ONE DAY AT A TIME

2022 DIARY

A Year-Long Journey of
Personal Healing and Transformation

Abby Wynne

GILL BOOKS

Gill Books

Hume Avenue

Park West

Dublin 12

www.gillbooks.ie

Gill Books is an imprint of M.H. Gill and Co.

© Abby Wynne 2022

978 0 7171 9208 3

All photographs courtesy iStock Photos and Unsplash.

Designed by Jane Matthews

Proofread by Susan McKeever

Printed by BZ Graf, Poland

This book is typeset in Neutraface.

A CIP catalogue record for this book is available from the British Library.

5 4 3 2 1

We are braver than we think, we can overcome
more than we expect and we will come through
much stronger for it. But we still need to walk
gently with compassion and kindness at the
forefront of our hearts, offering it to ourselves
and to each other.

To all of my readers, I wish for you a year where
you connect to an inner source of strength
and resilience. May you embody your learning
gracefully and painlessly as we continue together
on this path of growth and change, finding a new
respect for all living things and for this amazing
and beautiful planet upon which we live.

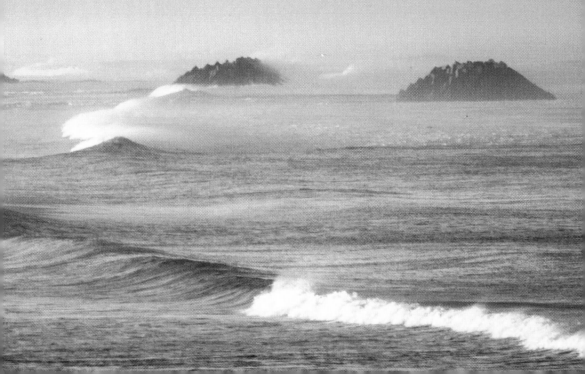

ABOUT THE AUTHOR

Abby Wynne is a bestselling Irish author and healer who blends shamanism, psychotherapy and energy healing to create a unique way of working, which she offers to the world through her books, online programmes and group healing sessions.

Abby's core teachings work towards empowering you to do your inner work with strength and courage while providing a structure and foundation to guide you. Abby also offers many other ways to feel supported while you are on your path of healing and empowerment, including downloadable healing audio files, healing jewellery and one-to-one sessions. Her Healing Circle also provides energetic support to its members on an ongoing basis.

You can join Abby on Facebook at Abby's Energy Healing Page, Instagram @abbynrghealing, Twitter @abbynrghealing or connect with her through her websites, www.abby-wynne.com or www.abbysonlineacademy.com.

Abby has made special downloadable files to go with this diary to enhance your healing experience. They are free, and you can find them on her website, www.abby-wynne.com.

'Much has been said about being in the present.
It's the place to be, according to the gurus,
like the latest club on the downtown scene,
but no one, it seems, is able to give you directions.'

BILLY COLLINS

Name ....

Address ....

Telephone ....

Emergency contact ....

USEFUL DATES

January
Saturday 1st ....New Year's Day

February
Tuesday 1st...St Brigid's Day

March
Thursday 17th..St Patrick's Day National Holiday

Sunday 20th ....Spring Equinox

April
Monday 18th ....Easter National Holiday

May
Monday 2nd ....May Public Holiday

June
Monday 6th ....June Public Holiday

Tuesday 21st...Summer Solstice

August
Monday 1st ....August Public Holiday

September
Thursday 22nd...Autumn Equinox

October
Monday 31st ....October Public Holiday

December
Wednesday 21st...Winter Solstice

Sunday 25th ....Christmas Day

Monday 26th...St Stephen's Day

Saturday 31st...New Year's Eve

THEMES FOR THIS YEAR

January...Love and Healing
February ....Peace and Stability
March ....Faith and Acceptance
April ....Inspiration and Balance
May...Spiritual Connection
June ....Purification and Self-Care
July...Grounding and Centring
August...Patience and Tolerance
September...Gratitude and Appreciation
October ....Grace and Authenticity
November ....Clarity and Focus
December ....Happiness

MOON PHASES CALENDAR
2022

January	2	●	9	◑	17	○	25	◐		
February	1	●	8	◑	167	○	23	◐		
March	2	●	10	◑	18	○	25	◐		
April	1	●	9	◑	16	○	23	◐	30	●
May	9	◐	16	○	22	◐	30	●		
June	7	◑	14	○	21	◐	29	●		
July	7	◑	13	○	20	◐	28	●		
August	5	◑	12	○	19	◐	27	●		
September	3	◑	10	○	17	◐	25	●		
October	3	◑	9	○	17	◐	25	●		
November	1	◑	8	○	16	◐	23	●	30	◑
December	8	○	16	◐	23	●	30	◐		

SPECIAL MOON EVENTS
2022

Saturday 30 April	Solar Eclipse
Monday 16 May	Lunar Eclipse
Tuesday 25 October	Solar Eclipse
Tuesday 8 November	Lunar Eclipse

CALENDAR
2022

JANUARY

Su	Mo	Tu	We	Th	Fr	Sa
						1
2	3	4	5	6	7	8
9	10	11	12	13	14	15
16	17	18	19	20	21	22
23	24	25	26	27	28	29
30	31					

FEBRUARY

Su	Mo	Tu	We	Th	Fr	Sa
		1	2	3	4	5
6	7	8	9	10	11	12
13	14	15	16	17	18	19
20	21	22	23	24	25	26
27	28					

MARCH

Su	Mo	Tu	We	Th	Fr	Sa
		1	2	3	4	5
6	7	8	9	10	11	12
13	14	15	16	17	18	19
20	21	22	23	24	25	26
27	28	29	30	31		

APRIL

Su	Mo	Tu	We	Th	Fr	Sa
					1	2
3	4	5	6	7	8	9
10	11	12	13	14	15	16
17	18	19	20	21	22	23
24	25	26	27	28	29	30

MAY

Su	Mo	Tu	We	Th	Fr	Sa
1	2	3	4	5	6	7
8	9	10	11	12	13	14
15	16	17	18	19	20	21
22	23	24	25	26	27	28
29	30	31				

JUNE

Su	Mo	Tu	We	Th	Fr	Sa
			1	2	3	4
5	6	7	8	9	10	11
12	13	14	15	16	17	18
19	20	21	22	23	24	25
26	27	28	29	30		

JULY

Su	Mo	Tu	We	Th	Fr	Sa
					1	2
3	4	5	6	7	8	9
10	11	12	13	14	15	16
17	18	19	20	21	22	23
24	25	26	27	28	29	30
31						

AUGUST

Su	Mo	Tu	We	Th	Fr	Sa
	1	2	3	4	5	6
7	8	9	10	11	12	13
14	15	16	17	18	19	20
21	22	23	24	25	26	27
28	29	30	31			

SEPTEMBER

Su	Mo	Tu	We	Th	Fr	Sa
				1	2	3
4	5	6	7	8	9	10
11	12	13	14	15	16	17
18	19	20	21	22	23	24
25	26	27	28	29	30	

OCTOBER

Su	Mo	Tu	We	Th	Fr	Sa
						1
2	3	4	5	6	7	8
9	10	11	12	13	14	15
16	17	18	19	20	21	22
23	24	25	26	27	28	29
30	31					

NOVEMBER

Su	Mo	Tu	We	Th	Fr	Sa
		1	2	3	4	5
6	7	8	9	10	11	12
13	14	15	16	17	18	19
20	21	22	23	24	25	26
27	28	29	30			

DECEMBER

Su	Mo	Tu	We	Th	Fr	Sa
				1	2	3
4	5	6	7	8	9	10
11	12	13	14	15	16	17
18	19	20	21	22	23	24
25	26	27	28	29	30	31

HOW TO USE THIS DIARY

There are several ways to use this diary; however you choose to use it is up to you. You can enjoy the flow of the graphics, the energy of the affirmations and quotes, and use the spaces to write down your appointments and to-do lists. Or you can use the energy of each month to inspire you and the writing space for journaling your thoughts and emotions. Think of this diary as a friend who reminds you to be nicer to yourself, encouraging you to take some time out for you.

This diary is designed to support you through the energy shifts of the coming year, through the monthly themes, exercises, affirmations and ways for you to go deeper. Again, it is up to you whether you spend time with this or not. Anything goes – there are no rules. I have written everything except for the 'going deeper' suggestions in the present tense to help bring you more into the present moment – this is a way to slow down, step out of time and reconnect to your heart. The more familiar you are with the words I use and the more you believe them to be true for you as you read them, the deeper the impact they will have on your healing process.

The basic premise of all my work is this: The relationship you have with yourself is the foundation of all your relationships. When you're kind to yourself, compassionate and at peace, you have a much more wholehearted life. Take it one day at a time – that's all any of us can do. Blessings to you on your healing journey this year.

THEMES

This diary will be able to travel with you through the ebbs and flows of emotional energy that you may experience as you move through the year. I have consulted with expert astrologists and have designed the themes around the coming astrological shifts, so that the diary will support you when times are difficult and enhance your ability for healing and growth wherever possible.

Try to take time at the beginning of each month to connect to that month's theme. Make time during the month to do the exercises. You are also free to look ahead to the coming months to prepare yourself. If you feel yourself coming out of balance, come back to the monthly invocation and reconnect. Reading the words out loud is much more powerful than reading them quietly to yourself. The affirmations are more powerful when you feel them deeply in your body, rather than just saying the words. They can help bring you back to your centre if you're feeling anxious or ungrounded. You can also replay the downloadable materials as often as you wish as additional support.

We are all different. We flow and change with time. One month you may delve deep, and another you may not – that's okay. If you choose to do the work that is offered here, to do it wholeheartedly you must do it your own way. Feel your way into it and you will know what is right for you. As time goes on, you will become more confident. A year is a long time, but it passes very quickly too.

At the end of each month, you are invited to reflect on how the month's theme impacted you. It's a way for you to mark the occasion and, over time, it's a good record of how far you have come on your healing journey. Using this diary gives you an opportunity to create, to dream and to grow, while tracking your progress throughout the year.

AFFIRMATIONS

Affirmations are statements of great meaning. I see them as a very powerful tool of transformation, if used with strong intention behind them. If you simply say an affirmation out loud, there is no power in it because you are just reading a group of words. However, if you take some time to bring your presence inwards and feel the meaning and power behind each word in the affirmation, then the energy behind the affirmation changes, and it can change your energy too.

Being in alignment with an affirmation happens when your mind, your heart and your gut instinct all resonate with it. For example, 'I deserve to be happy' could be something your mind agrees with, but there may be a hidden belief somewhere in you that doesn't agree at all. This belief can keep sabotaging you, just when things seem to be going well for you in your life. Saying 'I deserve to be happy' without a depth of feeling is a lost opportunity for you to learn if you are actually in alignment with the affirmation or not. Learning that you're not in alignment is a great opportunity to heal the part of you that doesn't believe, so that you can transform it and it no longer remains an obstacle in your life.

Try this exercise – choose an affirmation out of the book right now. Open the diary at any page and see which affirmation jumps out at you. Read the words silently to yourself, then bring your awareness inwards. Now speak the affirmation out loud with emotion. Does it sound like you believe it? Say it again and notice what you're thinking. If the mind believes it, you'll be fine with it, but if it doesn't, you'll hear all the reasons why it's not true for you. That's great! This is about getting to know yourself better. Now say it again, only say it from your heart. Ask your heart whether it totally agrees with what you have just said. Listen to your emotional response – are you soft and open, or have you shut down? Say it again one more time with your awareness in your stomach, your gut instinct. Do you feel strong, peaceful and stable, or do you feel nervous, anxious and ungrounded?

There are no right or wrong answers – what is true for you is your truth, but sometimes our truth is based on old things we learned as children that are no longer valid for us as adults. Examining what you hold as truth is part of a healing process so that you can decide if it still is a truth for you, or if it's something you would like to do some work on.

The affirmations in this diary are not daily; in fact, most of them span several days. This is to give you time to really tune into them so you can learn which ones you are not in alignment with and take the time to become so, if you wish. Try to say the affirmations each day, several times a day, with meaning, and let them grow on you. Healing is not about forcing or pushing change, but creating a space for you to grow. You're already perfect as you are and, if you don't believe that, perhaps that's an affirmation you'd like to work with too.

EXERCISES

The exercises are designed to help you relax and come more into the moment, and to help you find balance and stability. Try each one more than once. As you settle into them and get used to the feeling of being more in the moment, you may find them more effective for you. Try the free audio downloads from my website if you are having trouble settling. Let my voice create a safe space for you where you can really let go and relax. You can put the audio files on your mobile device and then you can listen to them anytime, anywhere, for a ten-minute mindfulness break.

GOING DEEPER

Thinking, writing and visualising are all part of healing, but so is taking action. I have given you ways to go deeper with the healing work for each month, but you don't have to do any of them. If you have a different idea that suits you better, do that instead!

CHECKING IN

Every three months I will ask you to take some time out to contemplate what you've just been experiencing, so that you can come into alignment with it and recognise what you have learned. This is an optional activity, but it will deepen your experience of growth and healing with this diary.

WHAT TO WRITE

I totally understand that brand-new, beautifully crisp, clean pages can be off-putting when it comes to putting pen to paper. However, this is your diary, and that is what it is here for. You don't need to pressure yourself to get it perfect, and you don't need to write for an audience either. All you need to do is write a thought or a feeling, make a list, or keep track of your emotions. Fun ideas include using different-coloured pens, doodling with colouring pencils, or even writing how you feel in poetry. So smudge away, cross out stuff and mess up that pretty page, but get the words out there. Once you get started, the writing will flow.

It might help if you take a minute or two to slow down and bring your awareness inwards before you start your writing. Perhaps take some time to breathe and disconnect from whatever is pulling you out of the present moment. Use the space to write down what is distracting you, so you can tell your mind, 'Look, I know and I've written it down! So you can stop reminding me!' You could ask yourself, 'What do I need to know today?' and then listen to your inner wisdom and write that down, as if you're taking dictation from a wise friend who is speaking to you. You could also write down what went well for you that day and what didn't, so you can remember what you would prefer to do the next time.

You could also rewrite the affirmation for the day or write a new one where one isn't present. Use the diary to write about what you need to do to look after yourself, or simply write in your appointments and your plans.

If you want, you can use the following prompts and see where they lead you: Today I feel ... Today I know ... Today I believe ... Today I am ... Today I want ... Today I wish ...

You've got a whole year ahead of you, and lots of ideas and opportunities. Do them all, or do none of them! Above all, please be patient with yourself. It's all here for you. Take your time and use the diary in a way that feels right for you.

SETTING YOUR INTENTION

Setting an intention for the year is a very powerful thing to do. Some people like to choose a single word for the year as a general theme, such as empowerment, joy, connection or growth. I like to make it a little more specific by writing down a statement or a paragraph that I can come back to time and time again. The beauty of setting an intention is that it can change and grow as you change and grow. The power behind it comes with your awareness of it.

HERE'S AN EXAMPLE OF AN INTENTION FOR THE YEAR THAT YOU CAN USE, BUT IT IS BETTER IF YOU WRITE ONE YOURSELF.

This year I will give myself the benefit of the doubt. I will take the time and space that I need for myself and ensure that I am always grounded and centred before responding to the challenges of life. I give myself permission to grow and change, and to heal a little bit more each day.

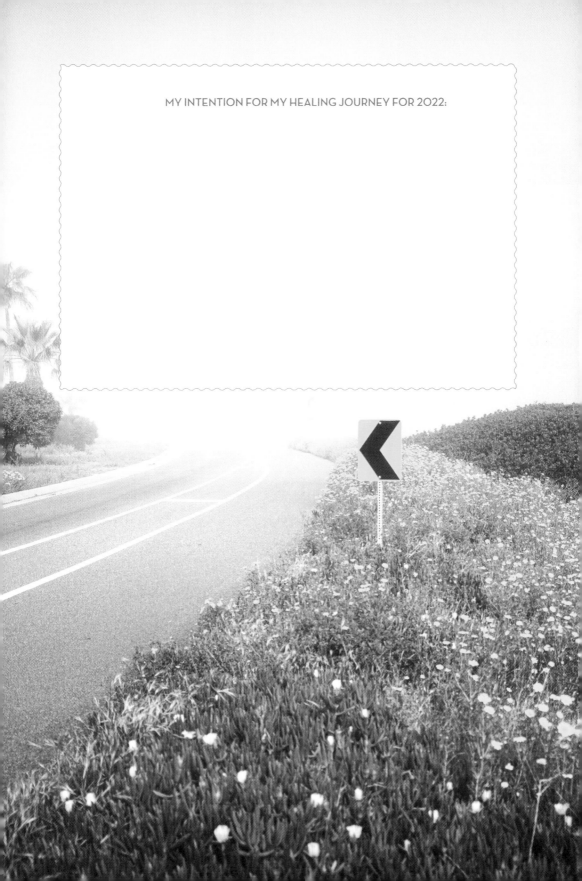

MY INTENTION FOR MY HEALING JOURNEY FOR 2022:

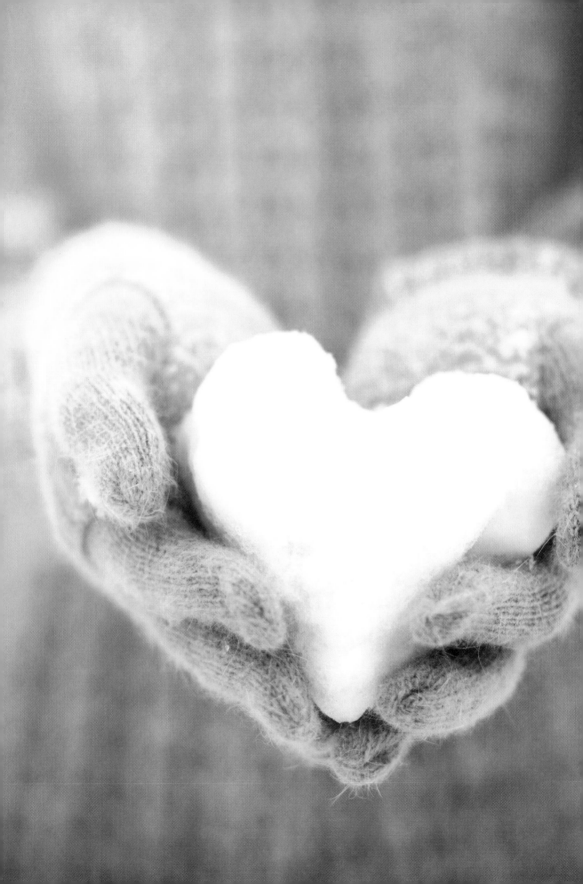

JANUARY

LOVE AND HEALING

**This year starts and ends with me,
and now I take my first step, one foot in
front of the other, one step at a time.**

'You're made of so much beauty, but it seems
that you forgot, when you decided that you were defined,
by all the things you're not.'

Erin Hanson

JANUARY

This year I will give myself the benefit of the doubt. I will meet myself where I am, change only the things that I can and learn how to love the rest. My life begins in this moment, right now. I cannot and will not wait for situations and things to be perfect before I let love and joy into my heart. Healing means letting go of all the things that are not me and becoming who I am in my wholeness. Perhaps there is nothing I actually need to fix; it's just how I think about myself that I need to change. I will let go of my expectations, meet life where it is and enjoy everything that is already here. I will meet myself where I am too. I open my heart to myself and pledge that, this year, I will treat myself well and learn how to accept myself and all the parts of myself completely.

EXERCISE

I close my eyes and breathe and slow down. I imagine I walk through a forest. When I am calm, I meet myself, exactly as I am right now. I look myself up and down and notice what I do not like. Then I notice what I do like. I look deeply into my own eyes and see that I'm truly doing the best I can. I feel my heart soften to myself. I will support myself. I know it's going to be alright.

GOING DEEPER

Make two lists – everything you like and everything you dislike about yourself. Walk away from them for a few hours and then come back. Look at what you dislike and ask yourself why you're so hard on yourself. Look at what you do like and spend some time appreciating yourself. What if you just let it all go and enjoyed yourself and your life for what it is? What is the worst thing that could happen?

SATURDAY 1

It is safe to give and to receive love

SUNDAY 2

MONDAY 3

I begin and end my day with peace

TUESDAY 4

WEDNESDAY 5

I breathe in love and I breathe out all that is not love

THURSDAY 6

FRIDAY 7

I deliberately fill everything I do with love

SATURDAY 8

I am compassionate and kind to myself

SUNDAY 9

I give permission for my heart to heal

MONDAY 10

I release all the obstacles between me and love

TUESDAY 11

I am learning how to love myself more

WEDNESDAY 12

THURSDAY 13

I let go of my need to be perfect

FRIDAY 14

I can meet myself where I am and support myself

SATURDAY 15

SUNDAY 16

I am not afraid to ask for help

MONDAY 17

I am learning how to be my own best friend

TUESDAY 18

WEDNESDAY 19

My body is doing the best it can with what I give to it

THURSDAY 20

I will learn how to treat myself better

FRIDAY 21

I open my eyes and am grateful for this and every day of my life

SATURDAY 22

Each day is an opportunity to let love in a little deeper

SUNDAY 23

MONDAY 24

I release anything in me that is afraid to love

TUESDAY 25

I surround myself with love

WEDNESDAY 26

I am learning how to look after myself

.

THURSDAY 27

I choose love, compassion and understanding

FRIDAY 28

I will never abandon myself

SATURDAY 29

I accept myself completely for who I am in this moment

SUNDAY 30

I thank the Universe for supporting me on my healing journey

MONDAY 31

Every day my light shines a little bit brighter

NOTES ON LOVE AND HEALING

Was this month's exercise useful to you?

Are your beliefs around the things you do not like about yourself based on fact or opinion?

Are your limiting beliefs based on your opinion or on someone else's?

How can you deconstruct these beliefs so that you can appreciate yourself more deeply?

FEBRUARY

PEACE AND STABILITY

**When there is peace in my heart,
there is peace in my world.**

'Not all those who wander are lost;
The old that is strong does not wither,
Deep roots are not reached by the frost.'

J.R.R. Tolkien

FEBRUARY

I want to accept myself at a deeper level. I am faced with a choice –
to continue this internal struggle or to let it go. I look around and notice
what is outside of me and what is out of balance. What emanates from
my being radiates outwards: peace starts from within. I must begin from
here. I relinquish my need for perfection and surrender this constant
battle with myself. The stillness of the world is here, in this moment, in my
heart. It feels good to soften to myself. When I soften, the world around
me softens too. This month I will notice if I take back up the struggle and
if so, I will endeavour to put it down again. Peace in every breath. Peace
in every step. Peace in my world. This is how I want to live now. Going
gently and leaving no footprints behind. I will learn how to walk this way,
at peace with myself, for the rest of my life.

EXERCISE

I breathe in peace. I breathe out everything that is not peace. I feel the
ground beneath my feet and I slow down. I breathe in peace and let go
of tension and urgency. I expand my energy and know that I have time for
everything I need to do. When I enlarge, I can hold and experience all of
my emotions. I soften to myself. I breathe in peace and breathe out all
that is not peace.

GOING DEEPER

Connect to nature. Spend time watching birds playing and water flowing. Play music
by Bach and wonder at the intricacies of the notes. Let the music hold you and
weave back together the fabric of your soul.

TUESDAY 1

May there be peace in my heart

WEDNESDAY 2

THURSDAY 3

It is safe to feel what I am feeling

FRIDAY 4

I can let go of big emotions

SATURDAY 5

I will do what I have to do to look after myself better

SUNDAY 6

With every step I soften to myself and the world

MONDAY 7

I let go of the things I cannot control

TUESDAY 8

I accept people where they are

WEDNESDAY 9

I accept myself where I am

THURSDAY 10

FRIDAY 11

I enjoy the feeling of stillness in my body and mind

SATURDAY 12

When I am still, I notice the beauty all around me

SUNDAY 13

When I expand, I have more tolerance for the world

MONDAY 14

The ground beneath me. The sky above me. I am held

TUESDAY 15

My day starts and ends with peace

WEDNESDAY 16

I slow down and connect to my heart

THURSDAY 17

FRIDAY 18

I am becoming my own best friend

SATURDAY 19

It is safe to experience all of my emotions

SUNDAY 20

I connect to a source of kindness and I am kind to myself

MONDAY 21

I move through the day with compassion and love

TUESDAY 22

I am learning how to accept myself completely

WEDNESDAY 23

I give myself the space I need to do the things I need to do

THURSDAY 24

I make my best choices when I consult my mind and my heart

FRIDAY 25

I take time out every day to connect to my inner wisdom

SATURDAY 26

I let go of other people's drama and emotional pain

SUNDAY 27

I no longer need to get tangled up to please someone else

MONDAY 28

I am good enough just as I am

REFLECTIONS ON FEBRUARY

Did you notice a difference in your body when you allowed yourself
to be still and let peace enter your heart?

_____

_____

_____

_____

_____

What changed for you? Can you notice more accurately
when you're moving out of a peaceful space?

_____

_____

_____

_____

_____

FAITH
AND
ACCEPTANCE

When I sit in stillness,
oceans of love enter my body
and I feel held.

'We feel most alive in the presence of the Beautiful,
for it meets the needs of our soul.'

John O'Donohue

MARCH

Our thoughts are subjective. They are influenced by our emotions and not necessarily the truth. I will never have all the answers. I can only have faith that what transcends this life, this world, is benevolent. It has my wellbeing at heart. I know that I am here to learn what I need to learn, to do the things that light me up and to spread love wherever I go. I open my heart to love and give myself permission to heal. I ask for peace to enter my heart and for my life to be in balance. This month I will trust that even though things may be difficult, I will get through them. I will be richer for the experience, even if it means my heart breaks open a little more, for the cracks are where the light gets in. I surrender to my growth process and ask a higher power to hold me safe in the palm of its hand.

EXERCISE

Imagine your heart has a door and that this door opens. Inside is a light. It's your inner light. Take a moment to visualise it – is it a tea light, a candle or perhaps a torch? Is it flickering or does it burn? With your kind, compassionate presence, does it burn brighter? Connect this light to the light of the sun and draw down a beam of light and sacred fire. Feel how this feels and trust that it is real. Understand that even on the darkest night or the dullest day, the sun is always there, even when you cannot see it.

GOING DEEPER

Spend some time in quiet contemplation. Read through the affirmations for this month and pick three that feel difficult to you. Sit with the reasons why. Ask yourself what you can do to work through them. Get some help if you need to. Work towards being able to say the affirmations and mean them 100 per cent.

TUESDAY 1

I know there is more to life than meets my eye

WEDNESDAY 2

THURSDAY 3

When I am quiet and still, I can feel the presence of love

FRIDAY 4

I can let go of how I think things are, and see them as they really are

SATURDAY 5

I can change or heal anything in me if I put my heart and mind into it

SUNDAY 6

MONDAY 7

What I want and what I need are not always the same thing

TUESDAY 8

I am willing to release my expectations of myself and of my life

WEDNESDAY 9

THURSDAY 10

I accept myself completely for who I am in this moment

FRIDAY 11

I can work with what I have right here and now

SATURDAY 12

I let go of my need to have things the way I want

SUNDAY 13

MONDAY 14

Today I will focus on supporting myself

TUESDAY 15

I ask the Universe to fill my heart with love

WEDNESDAY 16

I see the good in everyone, even those people I find difficult to be around

THURSDAY 17

I make space between me and the things that upset me

FRIDAY 18

I like the person that I am becoming

SATURDAY 19

SUNDAY 20

I believe in the good nature of people

MONDAY 21

When I am kind and generous, good things find their way back to me

TUESDAY 22

When I anchor my energy in the ground, I can allow myself to feel all of my emotions

WEDNESDAY 23

THURSDAY 24

Divine timing is not always my timing

FRIDAY 25

Every day I heal a little bit more

SATURDAY 26

I can give myself everything I need

SUNDAY 27

I make time to listen to my heart

MONDAY 28

I no longer need to cause myself emotional pain

TUESDAY 29

I am grateful for the lessons I am learning

WEDNESDAY 30

In my moments of stillness, I can feel the love that is here for me

THURSDAY 31

I bring my awareness into this moment and appreciate my life

NOTES ON FAITH AND ACCEPTANCE

What brought you the most peace this month?

How can you bring more peace into your everyday life?

CHECK IN

The themes for the first part of the year were Love and Healing,
Peace and Stability, Faith and Acceptance. The energetic signature of this year
so far has been difficult. Did you find that when you connected to love,
peace and faith, you were able to navigate the waves better?

Take some time right now to sit with all that you have learned
and all that you feel you have achieved. Well done.

....

....

....

....

....

....

....

—————————————————————————————

—————————————————————————————

—————————————————————————————

—————————————————————————————

—————————————————————————————

—————————————————————————————

—————————————————————————————

—————————————————————————————

Make sure to visit my website www.abby-wynne.com/onedayatatime
and sign up for my bonus recordings. You can also join me for an online energy
healing group session at the end of each calendar month if you would like more
support on your healing journey.

Now we move forward into the next three months of the year. Don't forget you
can revisit any of the affirmations or exercises of the past three months and
bring them with you as additional support.

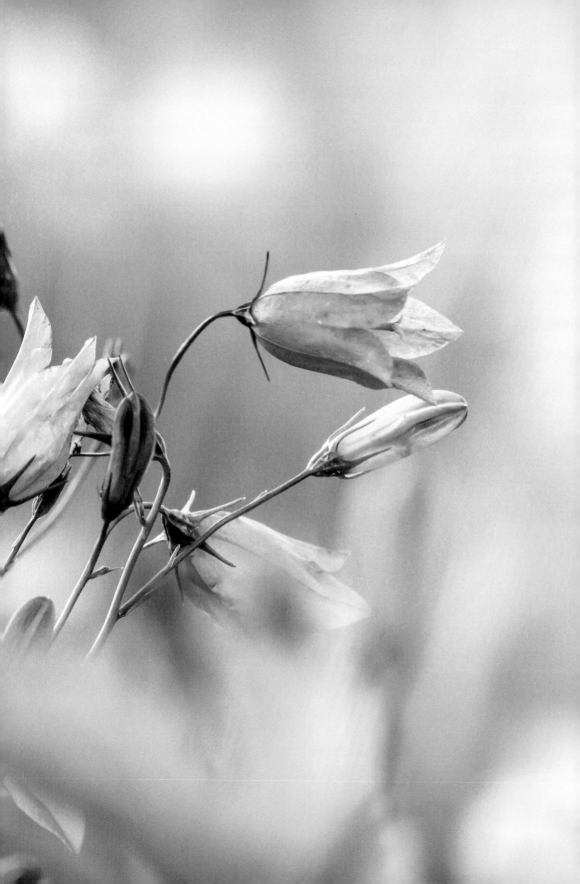

APRIL

INSPIRATION AND BALANCE

**My song builds up in my chest to be sung.
I must begin by singing it to myself.**

'For this soul needs to be honoured with a new dress woven
From green and blue things and arguments that cannot be proven.'

Patrick Kavanagh

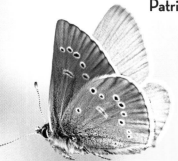

APRIL

I feel the year has finally begun. I have a freshness inside, a new awareness of myself and a lightness in my heart. My Soul longs to sing in a new language, with my new voice, yet I am shy to share my song with others. For now, I will find contentment in the details of my day and sing my song to myself. In quiet moments, in good company where I feel safe, I may whisper a verse or hum a bar or two. I know, deep in my centre, that this song is good because it's mine. It's still developing within me. I long to hear it. I will sing it loud and strong to myself. Just knowing it's there makes me stronger. When it's complete and bursting to come out into the world, I will set it free.

EXERCISE

I look at my face in the mirror and see the deeper layers beneath my skin. Layers of light, freshness and hopefulness for the world and for my life. I feel safe to be happy, to create and to shine my light to the world. When I feel anxious, I go to the part of myself that is in fear. I sit with it and ask it what it needs so that I can release the fear. I meet my own eyes in my reflection and smile. I know I can do this, for if I cannot live now, then when shall my life begin?

GOING DEEPER

You have changed. You may not realise to what extent, as this change has been accelerated. Spend some time in appreciation of how far you have come this year already. Look back on the past few months and appreciate all the work you have done. Don't forget to write your favourite affirmations in the first quarter check in.

FRIDAY 1

I am learning to like myself more

SATURDAY 2

SUNDAY 3

Not everyone will like me and that's okay, I do not have to like everyone in return

MONDAY 4

I deliberately choose things that make me happy

TUESDAY 5

I don't need to prove anything to anyone, including myself

WEDNESDAY 6

THURSDAY 7

I let go of my expectations and let love into my heart

FRIDAY 8

I can see what is good for me and I choose more of that

SATURDAY 9

I allow myself to look inside my own heart and see what is there

SUNDAY 10

Today I will be my own best friend

MONDAY 11

I give myself permission to shine my light in front of others without fear

TUESDAY 12

WEDNESDAY 13

THURSDAY 14

I no longer need to hide parts of myself to make other people happy

FRIDAY 15

I slow down and notice the details in the small things

SATURDAY 16

I can give myself a safe space to create my heart's desire

SUNDAY 17

I let go of my need for everything to be perfect

MONDAY 18

I listen to all sides and then I can make up my own mind

TUESDAY 19

WEDNESDAY 20

When I think too much, I turn the music on and dance

THURSDAY 21

I feel safe to experiment and make mistakes

FRIDAY 22

When I feel overwhelmed, I expand my energy and feel stronger

SATURDAY 23

I allow myself the freedom to express myself in the world

SUNDAY 24

I can spend time doing things that I love without guilt

MONDAY 25

Life is more fun when I put less pressure on myself

TUESDAY 26

I am allowed to make mistakes

WEDNESDAY 27

I treat myself well and I know how to look after myself

THURSDAY 28

I give myself permission to express my creativity

FRIDAY 29

I will let my heart lead me today

SATURDAY 30

I create from a place of joy and love

NOTES ON INSPIRATION AND BALANCE

Did you find you stopped yourself from being creative even when you were on your own?

Why do you think this was?

What can you do to support yourself so that you can break through

your blocks to expressing yourself?

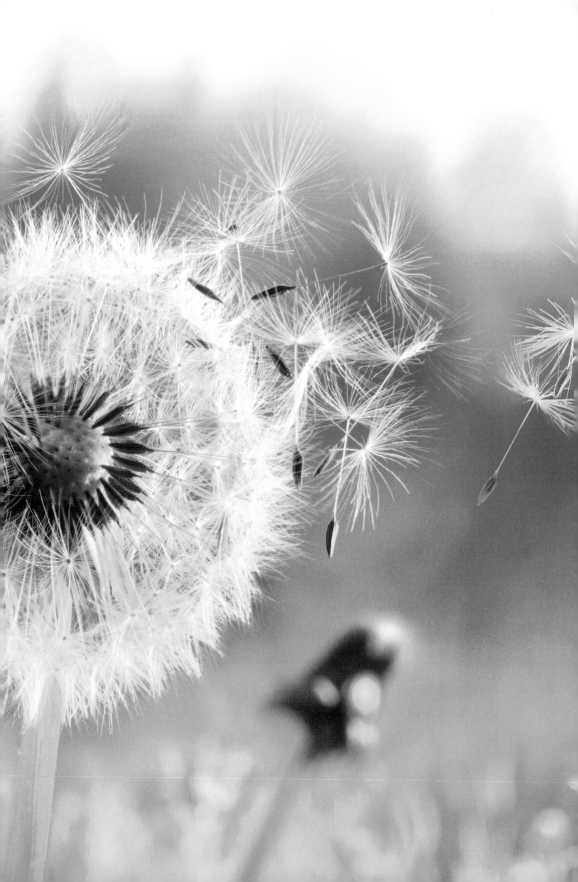

MAY

SPIRITUAL CONNECTION

**Woven into the fabric of everything
is a hidden light which shows itself
to those that know it is there.**

'The stars crawl onto my lap like soft animals
at night-time and God tucks my hair behind my ears
with the gentle fingers of her wind
and a new intimacy is uncovered in everything'

Chelan Harkin

MAY

When I slow my mind, detach from drama and connect to my heart, I feel the flow of life force energy in my body. It flows through me and out of me and into all things around me. I feel more connected to nature and to the source of all things. It's all too easy to lose this sensation. There is always something to pull me away from it and back into my thoughts. I realise this is a practice and that I need to bring my conscious awareness to it: when I do, I reap the rewards. When I'm outside and I disconnect from the day to day, I feel this connection become stronger. I will start from there. This month I'll take time each day to notice what is beautiful, to see the life force in everything, to feel it in myself and know that I'm part of something that's bigger than just me alone.

EXERCISE

Set an alarm for 10 minutes and turn off all distractions. Hand your troubles to the Universe so that you can focus. You can take your troubles back when the 10 minutes are over, if you want. Listen to the sounds that are around you. Feel the earth beneath you and the sky above you. Slow your thoughts. Imagine you are dissolving away, your body melting, so that nothing is left but your Spirit. You feel free, light and happy. You are held and you are loved. Let it in. Know that this is your true state of being.

GOING DEEPER

Do the exercise every day, where there are people, where there is busyness and where there is not. Do it more than once a day and do it often. Look at a flower and become the flower. Look at a tree and become the tree. When you imagine yourself dissolved, let the barriers you feel to love and to joy in your heart dissolve as well. Visualise yourself as a bright light shining, the energy of which burns away your stress and emotional pain. Take time to bring yourself back into the moment before you continue with your day.

SUNDAY 1

Every day I heal a little bit more

MONDAY 2

TUESDAY 3

When there is peace in my heart, there is peace in my world

WEDNESDAY 4

Today I will notice the beauty in everything

THURSDAY 5

I take time to feel the life force running through my body

FRIDAY 6

SATURDAY 7

I hand my troubles over to the Universe for safe keeping

SUNDAY 8

I will do all that I can, and that is enough

MONDAY 9

Every day I give myself space to connect with my Soul

TUESDAY 10

I grow towards the light

WEDNESDAY 11

I breathe in peace and breathe out all that is not peace

THURSDAY 12

FRIDAY 13

I am learning how to accept all of the parts of myself

SATURDAY 14

I forgive others and accept them where they are

SUNDAY 15

I am not afraid to speak out if I need to

MONDAY 16

TUESDAY 17

I take time to silence my mind

WEDNESDAY 18

I put a space between me and the things that encroach upon me

THURSDAY 19

There is time to do all of the things I need to do

FRIDAY 20

I make time to disconnect from the world and reconnect to my heart

SATURDAY 21

When I feel peace in my heart, I see peace in the world

SUNDAY 22

My day begins with peace and ends with peace

MONDAY 23

TUESDAY 24

I deliberately choose peace

WEDNESDAY 25

I give myself permission to release everything in me that is not at peace

THURSDAY 26

Today I will focus on filling my day with beauty, peace and love

FRIDAY 27

There is magic all around me

SATURDAY 28

I choose to fill my world with peace and love

SUNDAY 29

I expand my energy and make space in my heart for even more peace to come in

MONDAY 30

TUESDAY 31

I am completely at peace with myself

NOTES ON SPIRITUAL CONNECTION

REFLECTIONS ON MAY

What are the main things that distract you from being in the present moment?

....

....

....

....

....

How is your life different when you feel more connected to the moment,
to your heart and to the source of all things?

....

....

....

....

....

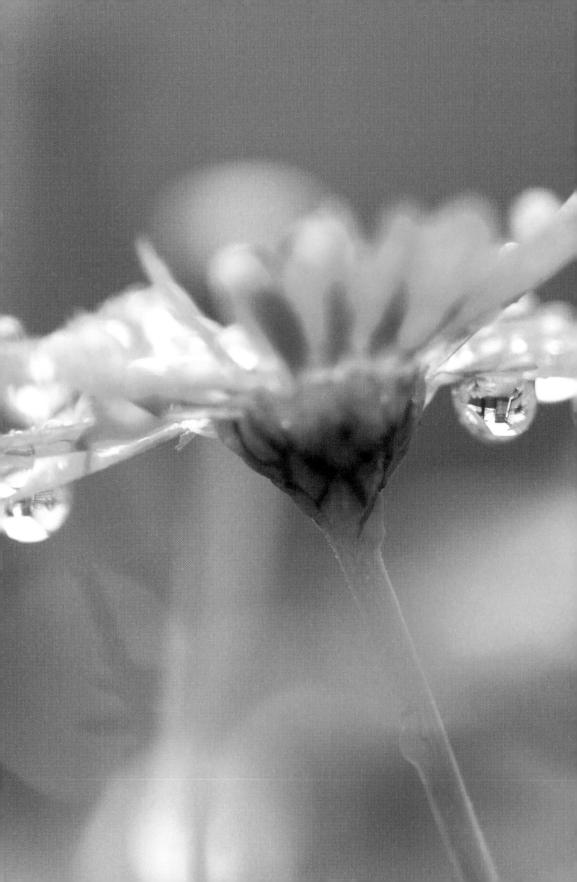

JUNE

PURIFICATION AND SELF-CARE

**I let go of everything that is not me
and allow myself to be filled
by the light of truth.**

'Then what I am afraid of comes. I live for a while in its sight.
What I fear in it leaves it, and the fear of it leaves me.
It sings, and I hear its song.'

Wendell Berry

JUNE

I stand in the river and let the waters wash me clean. I have lived for too long on other people's opinions, cutting off pieces of myself so that I fit in. Now is my opportunity to be who I am completely. I make peace with myself and all the parts of myself. I claim my space in the world. I let go of all the heaviness I am holding. I take the opportunity to turn a page, start again and give everyone the benefit of the doubt, including myself. I forgive but I do not need to forget. I promise myself I will look after myself better. I open my heart to compassion and kindness, to myself and to others. I'm not afraid to say no to things that are not good for me. I have good, strong, energetic boundaries. This month I will clear away what is no longer needed and move closer towards vibrant health.

EXERCISE

I imagine a crystal-clear waterfall with healing energies. I walk towards it in reverence. I choose what is heavy in me, loosen my grip upon it and let the waters wash it away. I feel lighter and whole. I remember who I am beneath the burden of my worries. I step out into the air and let the wind dry me, the sun warm me and the earth hold me. I am whole and new.

GOING DEEPER

Upgrade your level of self-care this month. Spend some time every day nurturing your body, mind and soul. Make an appointment for something nice to look forward to. Spend some time in nature or laughing with a friend, or both.

WEDNESDAY 1

I can look after myself

THURSDAY 2

FRIDAY 3

I can give myself everything I need

SATURDAY 4

I let go of what I want and trust that, if it is for me, it will come to me

SUNDAY 5

I allow grace and ease into my life

MONDAY 6

I appreciate my body and all that it does for me

TUESDAY 7

I let go of everything in the way of my vibrant health

WEDNESDAY 8

I have good, clear, strong boundaries

THURSDAY 9

FRIDAY 10

I allow myself to blossom and grow

SATURDAY 11

I breathe in beauty and breathe out all that is not beauty

SUNDAY 12

I have faith that the Universe is looking after me in perfect ways

MONDAY 13

What I want and what I need are not always the same thing

TUESDAY 14

I let go of all grudges that are holding me back from my best life

WEDNESDAY 15

I can say no to things with love in my heart

THURSDAY 16

FRIDAY 17

I know what is best for me and I do the right thing for myself

SATURDAY 18

I fill myself with love so that I have love to give

SUNDAY 19

I am enough just as I am

MONDAY 20

I give myself the time I need to make the changes I want to make

TUESDAY 21

I respect myself and only take on as much as I can handle

WEDNESDAY 22

I let go of my need to fix or change anyone or anything

THURSDAY 23

FRIDAY 24

I pull myself out of the situation and come back to myself

SATURDAY 25

I slow down and choose peace in every situation

SUNDAY 26

MONDAY 27

I don't need to compare myself to anyone else

TUESDAY 28

It is safe for me to feel what I am feeling

WEDNESDAY 29

I move through the day with compassion and love

THURSDAY 30

I am learning how to accept myself completely

NOTES ON PURIFICATION AND SELF-CARE

REFLECTIONS ON JUNE

What did you have the most trouble with this month and why?

....

....

....

....

....

How can you support yourself while continuing to do your healing work?

....

....

....

....

....

....

SECOND QUARTER OF THE YEAR
CHECK IN

These past few months we experienced themes of Inspiration and Balance,
Spiritual Connection, Purification and Self-Care. You have done a lot of work,
some of it very deep, which may have long-lasting effects on your life.

Take some time right now to sit with all that you have learned
and all that you feel you have achieved. Well done.

What do you feel was the biggest lesson of the past three months?

_____

_____

_____

_____

What was the most difficult thing you learned? How did you look after yourself?

_____

_____

_____

_____

How do you plan to move forward and embody all that you have learned?

....

....

....

....

....

Go back through the diary and choose your favourite affirmation, the one from the past
three months that made the most difference to you. Write it here for safe keeping.

....

....

....

....

Now we move into the second half of the year. If you are still doing the work of the last
three months, know that you must do your healing at your own pace and feel free to refer
back to the affirmations here.

Don't forget you can visit my websites www.abby-wynne.com and
www.abbysonlineacademy.com for downloadable meditations, energy healing
sessions, healing programmes and energy wisdom to support you on your journey.

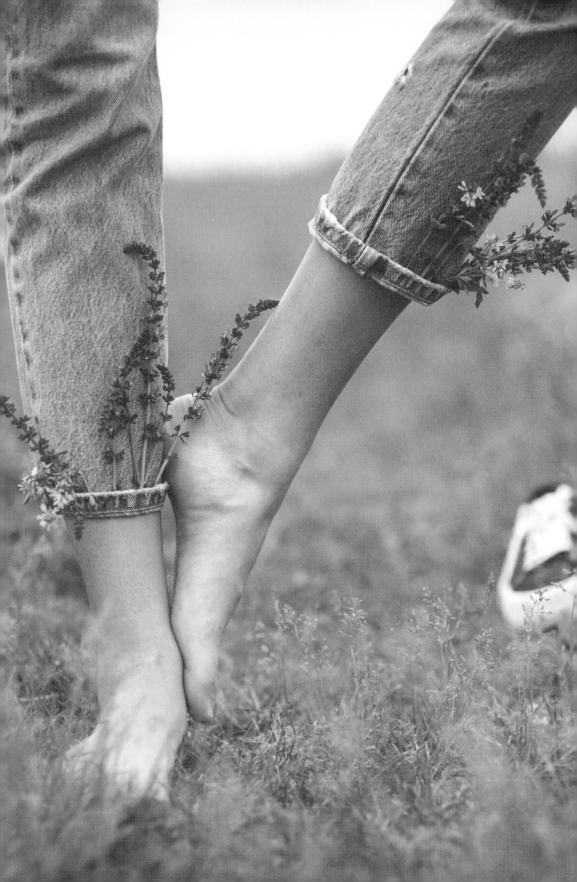

GROUNDING AND CENTRING

**I feel the ground beneath my feet.
I am here. I am safe.**

'Mountains never meet each other. Strong,
silent, rooted, they stay where they were planted,
gathering their strength. On difficult days, dissolve
your difficult thoughts. Become the mountain.'

A.W.

JULY

When the world spins too quickly for me, I know I need to slow down.
I ask my heart to help me. I know that what I fear is just a thought
and that in reality I am safe. I breathe and slow down and get my
bearings once more. I bring my presence deeper into my body with
every breath. I feel my feet inside my shoes and my shoes flat on the
ground. I grow roots deep down into the ground until I feel held. I slow
my breath and I relax. Then I look at the thought more clearly and
realise that it may not even be my own. Fear is an energy that looks for
weakness. Once it finds a weakness, it enters and takes over. I gather
my boundaries and push the thought and the energy away. I will do
what I need to do to look after myself this month.

EXERCISE

As stated in the invocation above, fear can be both inside and outside
of you. Read the words again and follow the instructions. Grow your
roots wide and deep until you feel stronger, and then push the fear
away. Once you're left with just the thought, you can choose how to
move forward.

GOING DEEPER

Make a list of everything that scares you. Share it with a friend. Make a plan and
clear each item off the list one by one until there is nothing you are unfamiliar with.
This is difficult work but it will make you stronger.

FRIDAY 1

I ask my power to come back into my body now

SATURDAY 2

SUNDAY 3

I pull my energy out of things that are outside of me

MONDAY 4

When I support myself, I can get through anything

TUESDAY 5

I bring my awareness deep into my body

WEDNESDAY 6

THURSDAY 7

I grow roots and extend my branches to the sky

FRIDAY 8

When I am planted and anchored and rooted, I expand

SATURDAY 9

I enlarge myself and feel safe to experience my emotions

SUNDAY 10

I send my energetic roots deep into the earth

MONDAY 11

TUESDAY 12

I ask fear that is not mine to leave my body now

WEDNESDAY 13

Today I will focus on peace and love

THURSDAY 14

I detach from drama and come back into my heart

FRIDAY 15

Today I will take it one step at a time

SATURDAY 16

SUNDAY 17

I let go of my worries and fears and choose love instead

MONDAY 18

I put a space of peace between myself and the rest of the world

TUESDAY 19

Love will get me through

WEDNESDAY 20

Today I will send love into everything, even things that are difficult

THURSDAY 21

When I make space for compassion, I make space for healing

FRIDAY 22

I breathe in peace and breathe out all that is not peace

SATURDAY 23

Everyone is doing the best they can with what they know at this time, including me

SUNDAY 24

I am ready to experience the joy/beauty/love that is here for me

MONDAY 25

I take time out to breathe and come back to myself

TUESDAY 26

WEDNESDAY 27

I anchor into the earth and unfold my energy outwards

THURSDAY 28

I am learning how to accept myself completely

FRIDAY 29

I am grateful for the lessons I am learning

SATURDAY 30

SUNDAY 31

I give myself the space I need to heal

NOTES ON GROUNDING AND CENTRING

REFLECTIONS ON JULY

Look back on the month and remember a difficult situation.
Think about when you felt grounded, and when you did not – what was different?

_____

_____

_____

_____

How will you remember to ground yourself the next time you feel uncentred?

_____

_____

_____

_____

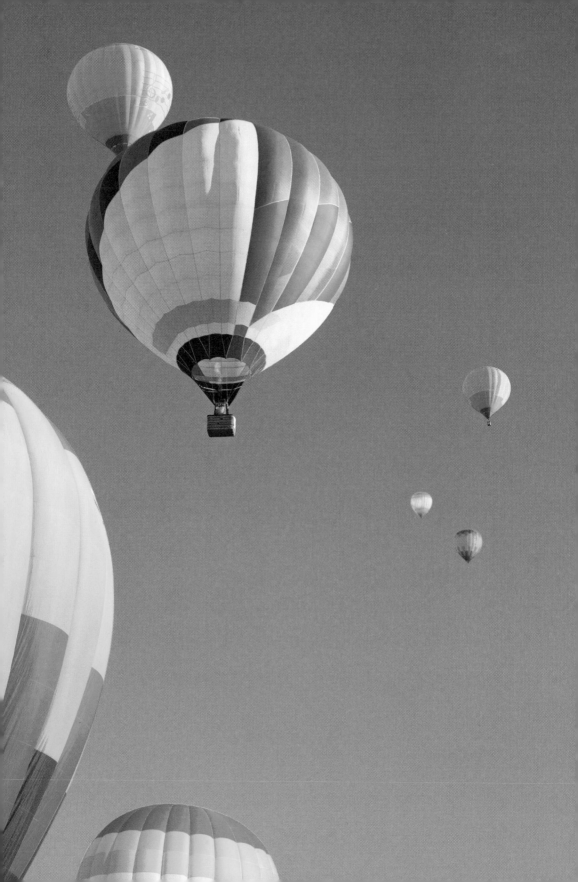

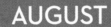

PATIENCE AND TOLERANCE

When I make space to breathe,
I find more patience and tolerance for myself,
and for the world.

'... you must accept change
before you die
but you will die anyway.
So you might as well live
and you might as well love.'

Pádraig Ó Tuama

AUGUST

When I get smaller energetically, I find that I get agitated and easily troubled.
I forget that I need to expand, I act out and I treat myself, and sometimes
others, badly. This month I'll focus on noticing this pattern in myself. When I
see it, I will be kind and gentle to myself, take a step back from whatever it is I
am engaging with and breathe. I've learned how to ground and centre myself;
I will start there. I've also learned how to bring peace into my heart, so I'll do
that next. Then I'll expand. When I take up space in the world, it's as if I push
the objects of my intolerance outwards and away from myself and create more
space for myself to breathe. Then I can see what I'm doing and I can let it go.
This month I'll look after my own needs first and then make space for others.

EXERCISE

I see myself as a shining ball of light. Everything that I'm connected to is
circling around me as if I'm the sun and they are the planets in my own
personal solar system. I slow down my thoughts and breathe, and then, when
I have peace in my heart, I push the planets further away from my centre, one
by one by one, until I feel like I have enough space for me.

GOING DEEPER

Clearing clutter in your home lets new, fresh energies come in. What are you
holding on to that you can let go of? What other types of clutter have you got
around you? You don't have to wait until spring to do a de-clutter. The energies
are good to do it now, so make space for something new and wonderful to
come into your life.

MONDAY 1

I create the space for new and beautiful things to come into my life

TUESDAY 2

I breathe and take a step away from what is irritating me

WEDNESDAY 3

I am grateful for my resistance and I find the learning there

THURSDAY 4

FRIDAY 5

I catch myself when I take things personally and then I let it go

SATURDAY 6

I no longer need to cause myself emotional pain

SUNDAY 7

I step away from drama, breathe, and reconnect to love

MONDAY 8

With love in my heart, I can say no to things that are not good for me

TUESDAY 9

WEDNESDAY 10

When I am patient with myself, I am patient with others

THURSDAY 11

I take the time I need to do the things I need to do

FRIDAY 12

I slow down and breathe, and expand until I feel more like myself again

SATURDAY 13

I am kind and patient towards myself and others

SUNDAY 14

I meet others where they are, and I meet myself where I am

MONDAY 15

I let go of my need to control

TUESDAY 16

WEDNESDAY 17

I find peace in the spaces in between

THURSDAY 18

When I am in the present moment, my presence fills me with patience and love

FRIDAY 19

SATURDAY 20

I deliberately choose love in every moment

SUNDAY 21

With kindness and compassion in my heart for myself, I have more tolerance for all

MONDAY 22

Kindness is at my centre, today I fill the world with kindness

TUESDAY 23

WEDNESDAY 24

With every step I take, I heal a little bit more

THURSDAY 25

I cannot see the big picture right now, so I will step back and trust the process

FRIDAY 26

SATURDAY 27

I ask for the strength that I need to get through the day/week/month

SUNDAY 28

I am grateful for everything that is going well in my life

MONDAY 29

I allow myself to feel all of my emotions

TUESDAY 30

I can see the good things all around me

WEDNESDAY 31

I choose to focus on beauty today

NOTES ON PATIENCE AND TOLERANCE

What was the most difficult affirmation for you to come into
alignment with this month and why?

....

....

....

....

....

List your 3 biggest triggers. How can you protect yourself around
being triggered in the future?

....

....

....

....

....

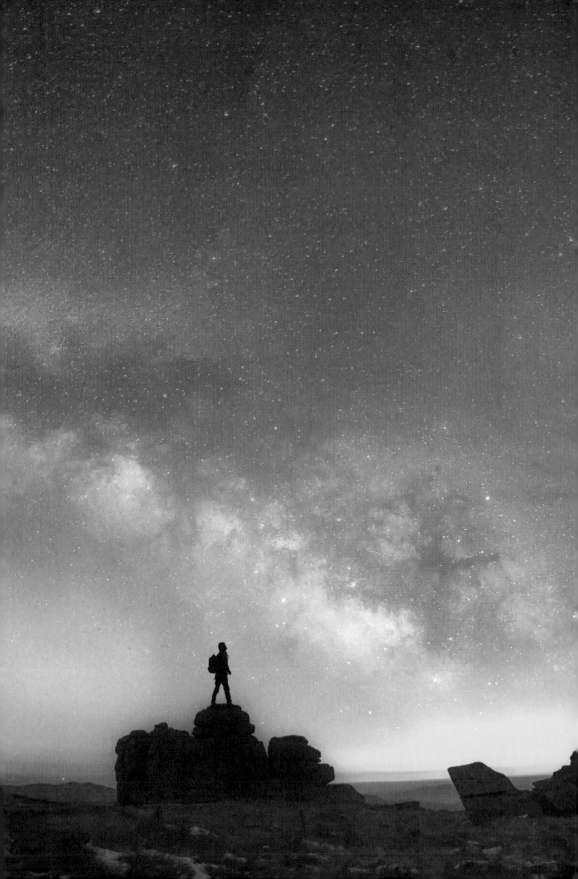

GRATITUDE AND APPRECIATION

I have let go of my inner struggle
and am enjoying life more deeply
as I become my own best friend.

'Better just to assume that you are never more than
one moment old, and your body is made of stars
so ancient their light is arriving only now.'

Alfred LaMotte

SEPTEMBER

I look around myself at my life. I look at the work I have done and the people I care about. I appreciate everything that's here. I know I can find patience to fix the things I'm still not happy with. I'm truly grateful for everything in my life. I know I'm still a work in progress and that there's more learning and healing to do. I'm happy knowing that I'm doing my best and that every day I'm a little more at peace. I'm becoming my best healed self. I'm allowed to get angry. I'm allowed to feel all of my emotions. I no longer try to fit in and please others before I please myself. I'm finding an inner strength that I did not know I had. I notice more and more that when I look to others for the answers I need, I can become ungrounded. I'm grateful that I know how to disconnect from the outside world and reconnect to me.

EXERCISE

Keep a gratitude journal this month – you can use this diary if you want. Each night before you go to bed, list five things that you are grateful for. Each item must be different; never repeat the same thing twice. At the end of the month, read back through everything you have written. Absorb the positive energy and marvel at the beauty you have around you.

GOING DEEPER

I imagine that I am a ball of light. I see cords and tentacles of light stretching outwards from my centre and wrapping around things that drain my energy, things I think I need to know the answers for and things that I am worried about. I see my energetic tentacles loosen their grip and unwrap themselves. I pull them back into me. I feel more centred and grounded when I am here, in this moment. I let it all go and appreciate everything for what it already is.

THURSDAY 1

I experience the world through loving eyes

FRIDAY 2

I give myself permission to release everything in me that is not at peace

SATURDAY 3

I am grateful for the things that I have in my life and the things that are yet to come

SUNDAY 4

MONDAY 5

I open my heart to love and I allow love into my life

TUESDAY 6

I am grateful for the beauty that surrounds me

WEDNESDAY 7

I accept myself completely for who I am

THURSDAY 8

I am grateful to be in the flow of life

FRIDAY 9

SATURDAY 10

I am filled with joy and appreciation for the potential in my life

SUNDAY 11

I am learning how to be my best, healed self

MONDAY 12

When I deliberately connect to a source of love, I feel happy and content

TUESDAY 13

I respect all human beings no matter where they are on their journey

WEDNESDAY 14

I am grateful for my body and all the work that it does for me

THURSDAY 15

I am grateful for my voice and that I can say what I need to say

FRIDAY 16

SATURDAY 17

I am grateful for all of my emotions as within them lies the richness of life

SUNDAY 18

There can be beauty in difficult situations

MONDAY 19

I trust in my intuition and I make good choices

TUESDAY 20

I slow down and take time to let beauty into my life

WEDNESDAY 21

I open my heart to love and joy and I let life inspire me

THURSDAY 22

I trust that the Universe is looking after me in perfect ways

FRIDAY 23

I am grateful for my mind and how it supports me and looks after my needs

SATURDAY 24

I relish the smells, sounds, colours and tastes that I experience

SUNDAY 25

I am grateful for the opportunities that I experienced this year

MONDAY 26

TUESDAY 27

I forgive myself completely for everything I have or have not done

WEDNESDAY 28

I give myself and others the benefit of the doubt

THURSDAY 29

I give myself permission to be happy and at peace

FRIDAY 30

NOTES ON GRATITUDE AND APPRECIATION

REFLECTIONS ON SEPTEMBER

How did it feel to read out your gratitude lists at the end of this month?

What was the theme that kept repeating itself in your lists?

....

....

....

....

You can continue to write lists as a bedtime ritual if you enjoyed doing it.

Make a list now of the top 20 things that you appreciated most this month.

....

....

....

....

....

....

CHECK IN

During the past few months we experienced themes of Authenticity and Vitality,
Presence and Beauty, Safety and Grounding. These are all big, strong themes.
Which one affected you the most?

Do you feel you're able to look after yourself better,
based on the learning that you've already gained this year?

What do you feel was your greatest personal achievement during the past three months?

....

....

....

....

What was the most difficult experience? How did you look after yourself?

....

....

....

....

Go back through the diary and choose the affirmations that made the most difference to you in the past three months. Write them here for safe keeping.

....

....

....

....

....

....

....

Go to my website, www.abby-wynne.com/onedayatatime, and make sure you have signed up for my bonus recordings. Perhaps you'd like to take some time to listen to a few of the visualisations and meditations to consolidate what you have done so far this year.

Now we move into the last three months of the year. Know that you must do your healing at your own pace, so feel free to revisit any of the previous themes in the diary and carry the energy of those affirmations into the coming months.

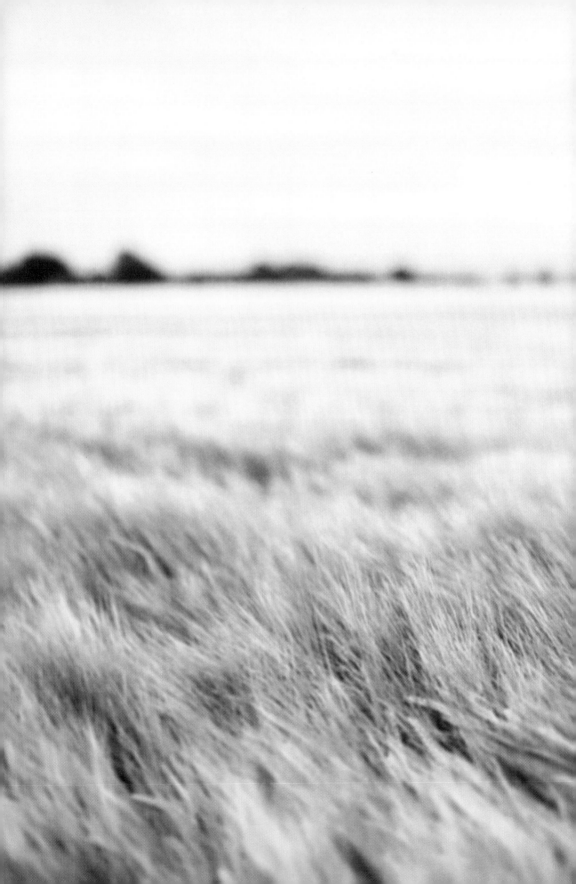

OCTOBER

GRACE AND AUTHENTICITY

I shine my light and sing my song. I am alive and this is my one and only life.

'I dreamt ... that I had a beehive here inside my heart.
And the golden bees were making white combs
and sweet honey from my old failures.'

Antonio Machado

OCTOBER

When I let go of my fixed ideas, I look at the world anew with the eyes of
a child and I have a new appreciation for life. When I am still, I see the life
force flowing through everything. I am feeling lighter and happier after my
month of gratitude. I let go of my need to hide, to please others and to stay
in the shadows. I can be real. I can be unapologetically me and unafraid to
speak my truth. This year I have expanded. I'm learning my song and I'm
getting ready to sing it out loud. There's so much beauty in the world. I'm
learning the connection between gratitude, truth, beauty and grace. I can
find grace in everything, even things I once thought were ugly. I'm able to
find grace and beauty in myself too and this has changed everything for me.
I am ready to offer my light to the world, to be of service to others, while
always looking after myself.

EXERCISE

I bring my awareness into my body and breathe. I slow down and imagine
I grow roots into the ground. I breathe in the nourishing energy of Mother
Earth. I sense a ball of healing light above my head. It drops a cord of light
into me and I breathe it down and into my body. This light fills me with
peace, joy and love. With every breath in, I breathe in healing light. With
every breath out, I let go of all that I am not.

GOING DEEPER

You can listen to many healing audios from Abby's Online Academy if you want
to immerse yourself in healing energies this month. Spend some time listening to
things that uplift you, look at the world with eyes of wonder and continue your
gratitude list from September if you want to. It is completely up to you!

SATURDAY 1

When I am patient with myself, I am more patient with others

SUNDAY 2

I am not my thoughts, I am not my emotions, I am the shining light beneath

MONDAY 3

I no longer need to cause myself emotional pain

TUESDAY 4

WEDNESDAY 5

I forgive myself for everything I have or have not done in my life

THURSDAY 6

I bring more of my presence into the world

FRIDAY 7

I release all of the pressure that I put upon myself

SATURDAY 8

I make the time to quiet my mind and listen to my inner wisdom

SUNDAY 9

MONDAY 10

I feel the earth beneath me and the sky above me and I feel held

TUESDAY 11

When I connect to the earth, I feel calmer and more centred

WEDNESDAY 12

I am free to completely be who I am in this moment

THURSDAY 13

I hand my troubles over to the Universe for safe keeping

FRIDAY 14

I slow down and make space for what it is that I am feeling today

SATURDAY 15

I take the time I need each day to reconnect to my heart

SUNDAY 16

MONDAY 17

I have good, strong, energetic boundaries

TUESDAY 18

I separate my mind from my heart and listen to each in turn

WEDNESDAY 19

I allow myself to express myself in many different and creative ways

THURSDAY 20

I slow down and bring myself into the present moment

FRIDAY 21

I am able to look after myself

SATURDAY 22

Today I connect to a source of unconditional love

SUNDAY 23

MONDAY 24

I do not need to fix or change anything

TUESDAY 25

I move through the day with compassion and love

WEDNESDAY 26

THURSDAY 27

I am kind and gentle to myself

FRIDAY 28

I forgive myself for the mistakes that I have made

SATURDAY 29

SUNDAY 30

I allow myself to let go of anger and emotional pain

MONDAY 31

I feel strengthened and encouraged by the possibilities in my life

NOTES ON GRACE AND AUTHENTICITY

Think about a time in your life when you felt bright and happy – how old were you?
What was that like for you? Can you emulate that feeling now?

....

....

....

....

What's in the way of you being happy now? How can you release it?

....

....

....

....

....

....

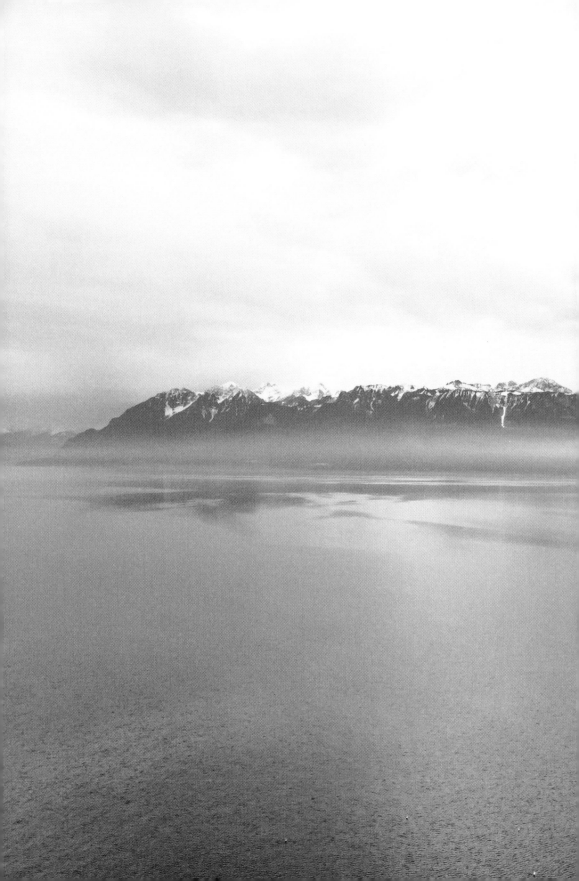

CLARITY AND FOCUS

The quality of my life depends on the quality
of my thoughts, and the quality of what
I choose in every moment.

'This whole thing is ridiculous – spending an enormous amount
of energy searching for love – Isn't every single fibre in your
being spun from the energy of love?'

Guthema Roba

NOVEMBER

My mind is clear. I know who I am. I'll spend this month integrating all of the work I've done this year. I'll use this diary to help me and I'll get outside help if I need it. I'm certain that I want a happy life and I'm strong enough to pinpoint where I'm still having trouble with my inner work, even if I'm not sure exactly what the issue is. I pledge that I'll become more aware of my thoughts, make better choices and start a process that will take as long as it will take to raise the overall quality of my life. I'm patient and tolerant with myself, I accept myself completely and I set the ball rolling, without needing it to be perfect right now. It's possible that all I need to do is change a fixed way of thinking. Perhaps everything is already perfect and I'm just not seeing it yet. I'll take this month to find out.

EXERCISE

I choose an affirmation from this diary that resonates with me. I say it out loud and mean it 100 per cent. I say it once more, bringing my awareness deep into my heart. I repeat it until my heart opens and I mean it 100 per cent. I bring it down into my stomach and say it out loud once again. I let go of the fear of being completely myself. I like myself more and more each day. Now is my time to live fully in the present moment.

GOING DEEPER

Find another affirmation from the diary that you have had trouble with up to this point but want to fully resonate with. Sit with it and try to understand what is troubling you around it – is it a limiting belief from your childhood? Are you ready now to let it go? Get some help if you need to, unlearn the toxic thoughts that no longer serve you and replace them with the medicine of the affirmations instead.

TUESDAY 1

I trust my inner wisdom and give myself the things I need

WEDNESDAY 2

THURSDAY 3

I invite light into my life and I open my heart to love

FRIDAY 4

I will make time to look at what isn't working for me, and learn what is the root cause

SATURDAY 5

I am not afraid to ask for help

SUNDAY 6

I surround myself with people and things that fill me with love

MONDAY 7

I am able to say no to things with love in my heart

TUESDAY 8

I am loving and kind to myself and others

WEDNESDAY 9

I release all judgements and see the world through compassionate eyes

THURSDAY 10

I can let go of things that I wasn't able to let go of before

FRIDAY 11

SATURDAY 12

I am safe, I am strong, and I am here

SUNDAY 13

Giving myself what I need is self-care

MONDAY 14

I see myself and all that I have experienced and I appreciate how far I have come

TUESDAY 15

I give myself permission to take some time for me today

WEDNESDAY 16

THURSDAY 17

When I am kind to myself, I have more kindness to offer other people

FRIDAY 18

I am learning how to look after myself

SATURDAY 19

I will show up for myself and do what is needed

SUNDAY 20

When I support myself, I can overcome my fears

MONDAY 21

Just for today, I will release all of the pressure I put on myself

TUESDAY 22

Love softens all of my sharp edges

WEDNESDAY 23

I no longer need to criticise myself

THURSDAY 24

I am kind and compassionate to myself

FRIDAY 25

I like who I am right now, in this moment

SATURDAY 26

SUNDAY 27

I trust my inner wisdom and give myself the things I need

MONDAY 28

I release myself from unrealistic expectations

TUESDAY 29

I am free to be completely myself in every moment of every day without fear

WEDNESDAY 30

NOTES ON CLARITY AND FOCUS

Which affirmation from this diary is your favourite? Which is the most useful?

How do you use them in your life?

_____

_____

_____

_____

_____

Which affirmations do you still have trouble with?

What can you do to support yourself to work through your difficulties with them?

_____

_____

_____

_____

_____

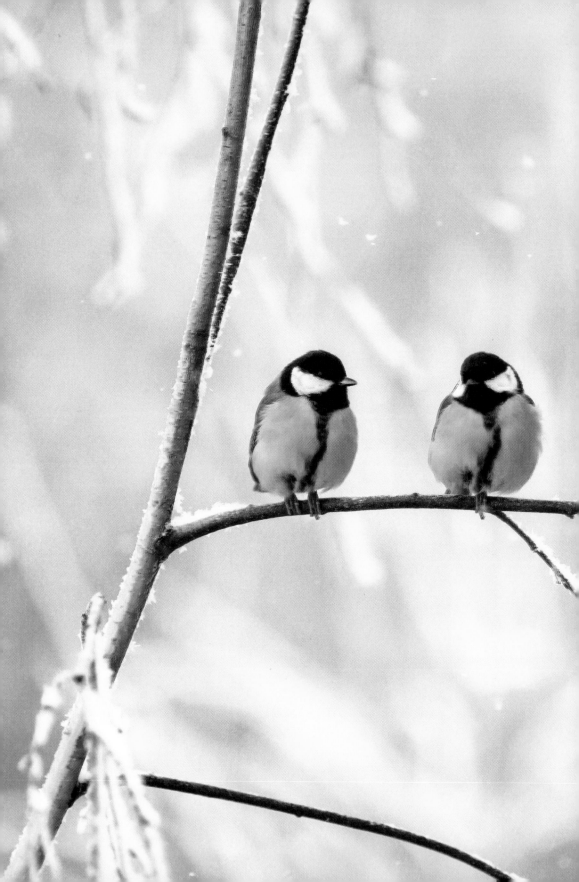

DECEMBER

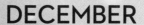

HAPPINESS

I am becoming the flower in bloom.
I do not need to chase the bee,
I let the bee come to me.

'I lie here in a riot of sunlight
watching the day break and the clouds flying.
Everything is going to be alright.'

Derek Mahon

DECEMBER

It's been a challenging year but I've come through it stronger and wiser. I'm authentic in how I speak and move in the world. I'm not afraid to say how I feel, even if it won't please everyone. I allow myself to try new things and I have a new appreciation for all the life around me. I'm kinder to myself and happier in my relationships. I imagine my happiest life and feel deep within that it's possible to have this now. When I'm strong in my centre, and grounded and expansive in my energies, I attract more of the things that I want. This month I celebrate my ability to bring more happiness into my own life. I celebrate a sense of freedom that I get to choose what I want more consciously. Being generous and kind no longer depletes my energy reserves. It is easy to love other people and I like myself more than I ever did before. I am now ready to rest and enjoy the gifts of the work I have done.

EXERCISE

I imagine that I am a radio. I tune into the station of happiness. I allow the energy of happiness to fill my body completely and I notice what happens to me when I do that. I bring my awareness to the parts of myself that are uncomfortable and reassure them with kindness and compassion. Little by little, the more I do this, the easier it gets. Happiness is my natural state. I am getting closer to feeling like this most of the time.

GOING DEEPER

To focus more on happiness, deliberately plan things that will uplift you. Spend time with people that you love, watch a movie that you enjoy or cook a dinner that you can share with a friend. Notice how much you enjoy the simple things, and how being generous and kind no longer depletes your energy reserves.

THURSDAY 1

When I am happy, I spread happiness wherever I go

FRIDAY 2

SATURDAY 3

The more kindness I give, the more it comes back to me

SUNDAY 4

I give myself permission to feel happy and free

MONDAY 5

I make good and healthy choices for my body, mind and soul

TUESDAY 6

I open myself to love and let love in

WEDNESDAY 7

I deliberately choose to focus on what makes me happy today

THURSDAY 8

My happiness does not depend on other people

FRIDAY 9

SATURDAY 10

I deliberately surround myself with beautiful things

SUNDAY 11

I give myself the space I need to process my difficult emotions

MONDAY 12

When I let go of things I no longer need, I make more space for joy

TUESDAY 13

WEDNESDAY 14

I breathe in deep, open my heart and drink from the beauty of life

THURSDAY 15

I can give myself anything I want

FRIDAY 16

I listen to my inner wisdom and do what I need to do

SATURDAY 17

I choose to create my life from a place of love

SUNDAY 18

I accept myself completely as I am

MONDAY 19

TUESDAY 20

I let go of anything that stands in the way of my happy life

WEDNESDAY 21

I am not afraid to make mistakes

THURSDAY 22

I am grateful for all of the happiness that lives inside of me

FRIDAY 23

I slow down and breathe and connect to an inner source of happiness

SATURDAY 24

I pull all of my energy out from things outside of me and call it back into me

SUNDAY 25

I find happiness in small things

MONDAY 26

TUESDAY 27

I let go of my need to control, and trust that everything is as it should be

WEDNESDAY 28

I release the things I no longer need, and I welcome joy into my heart

THURSDAY 29

I stop and breathe and see the world through loving eyes

FRIDAY 30

SATURDAY 31

I breathe in love and breathe out all that is not love

NOTES ON HAPPINESS

What would it be like for you to live your best and happiest life, now?

....

....

....

....

....

How can you look after yourself during the holidays and into the coming year?

....

....

....

....

....

FINAL QUARTER OF THE YEAR
REFLECTIONS

The last three themes were Grace and Authenticity, Clarity and Focus, and Happiness. It's wonderful to end the year on a happy note. What was it like for you to move from difficult energies into high-vibrational grace, love and gratitude? Did you feel any differences in your body? How are you feeling now? Take some time right now to sit with all that you have learned and all that you feel you have achieved. Well done.

What do you feel was your greatest moment this year?

What was the most difficult? How did you look after yourself?

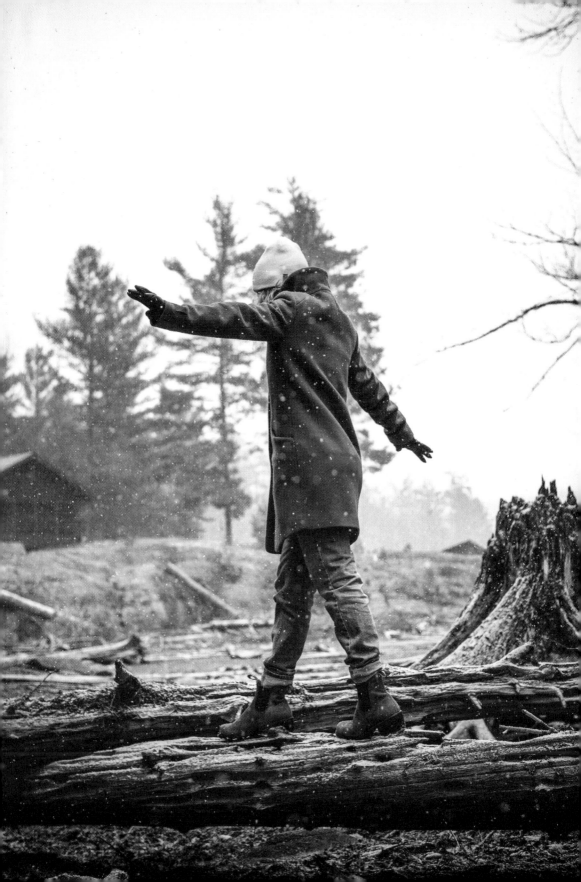

REFLECTIONS
2022

What do you wish for yourself for 2023? Take a moment to get in tune with yourself, and then write it down to clarify it for yourself.

_____

_____

_____

_____

_____

_____

_____

_____

_____

If you'd like to keep travelling with the *One Day at a Time Diary*, you can purchase the new diary either online via my website, or in any Irish bookshop. I hope that it was a useful guide and support to you over the past 12 months.

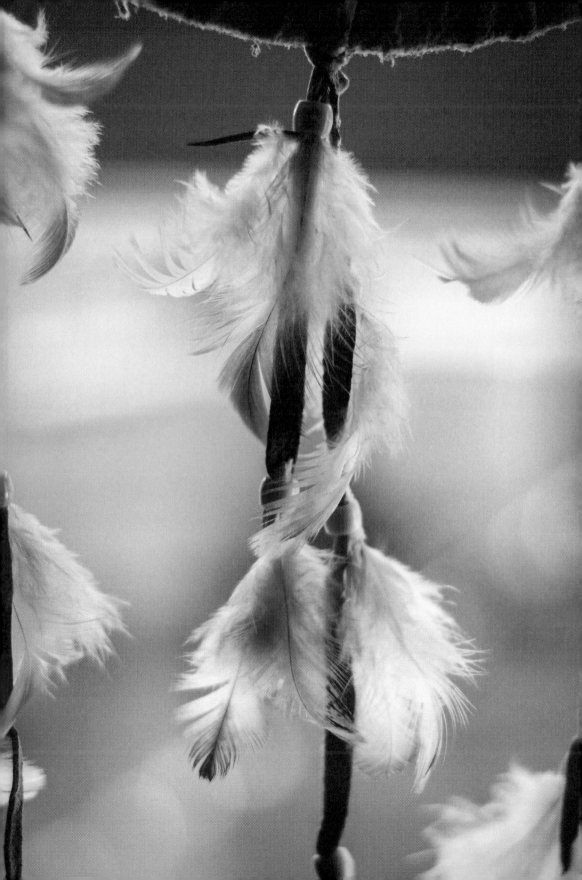

ACKNOWLEDGEMENTS

Gratitude to Sarah Liddy, commissioning editor; Rachael Kilduff, Teresa Daly and Jane Matthews, for being such a great team to work with. I'd also like to thank Ellen Monnelly for her continued support with my social media campaigns and publicity, and Paul Neilan for always answering my sales queries so promptly! I also want to thank everyone at Gill Books who worked hard behind the scenes to get yet another fabulous diary out into the world.

Deep appreciation and gratitude to my inner circle of friends and loved ones, to my healing guides and to my family. And, of course, to my dear readers who are loyal and brave and show up and do their inner work. I see you and I salute you all.